Eating Disorder Recovery Handbook
Lize Brittin
Edited by Kevin Beck

.

* * *

* * *

TABLE OF CONTENTS

* * *

Introduction

"There is no magic cure, no making it all go away forever. There are only small steps upward; an easier day, an unexpected laugh, a mirror that doesn't matter anymore." -- Laurie Halse Anderson

When I first started writing my memoir *Training on Empty*, it was partly to tell my personal story but mainly to offer hope and inspiration. I wanted to show others that recovery from anorexia and other eating disorders is possible.

Not long after I wrote the book, I started a companion blog. As I have continued to build this over the years, I discovered anew that recovery is a process. Every year, I grow and learn new lessons. Recovery, a bona fide full recovery, is possible, but it takes staying one step ahead of the illness. It requires recognizing patterns and triggers, and finding new coping strategies in order to stay healthy. Most of all, it takes radical trust in yourself and total self-respect to truly get over an eating disorder.

For over 20 years, I struggled with an eating disorder, primarily anorexia. It was a severe case, one that nearly killed me, and I spent time in hospitals, went to therapists, read books and even tried countless alternative therapies, all in an effort to overcome my illness and mostly in vain, though I can't discount all I was able to take in along the way. I felt like I was on a quest for a magic pill. I was looking for answers outside myself, sure that something or someone could make me feel better.

The more the illness consumed me, the more frantic and concerned my friends and family became. Their emotions ranged from frustration and anger to sadness. On some level, I understood that, in a way, I was choosing this agony, much like an alcoholic chooses to drink, but I felt completely stuck, unable to help myself. I knew there was a way out of the hell I was creating, but I couldn't see how to free myself. I felt like I was in prison, but people kept saying I had put myself there. How could this be? On an intellectual level, I knew what I needed to do to get well, but I couldn't seem to make a move, any move, in the right direction.

My mom, who had overcome terrible hardship in her life, kept telling me that in order to recover, I had to want to get well, really want it. The results of the changes I envisioned were appealing, but putting them in place seemed impossible. It meant letting go of certain behaviors, my unhealthy coping mechanisms. Food to me was never really related to hunger. Early in my life, I ate for comfort. Later, I restricted to gain a sense of control in what felt like a stressful environment. My eating disorder was like a security blanket, a deadly one.

In her book, "Eating in the Light of the Moon", Dr. Anita Johnston offers a wonderful analogy. She describes a scene in which a girl is struggling after falling into a river and gets swept downstream. She is overwhelmed and can't swim to shore. In a frantic effort to survive, the girl grabs onto a log. This log keeps her afloat, but it's also pulling her further down the river. Meanwhile, people on the banks of the river see a simple solution: let go and swim to shore. The people shout at her to let go and swim, but she's too afraid to let go. She has convinced herself that she needs the log. It did initially save her, after all. The problem is that the floating lumber is now carrying her away and may eventually take her into dangerous waters that will ultimately drown her.

Obviously the log in the story represents the addiction or disorder we choose in order to cope. It can be addiction, eating issues, bad relationships or any coping method that isn't healthy. It serves us in the short term in the sense that it offers us a way to feel like we are surviving in a chaotic situation, but it's not a comfortable way to live. In fact, it may kill us in the end.

For anyone struggling with these issues, it's important to ask what purpose the illness or addiction has served. What does having the disorder keep you from experiencing? Why are you drawn to the disorder, and what security does the illness provide and at what expense? It's impossible to swim to shore without strength.

Coping not only takes courage but also a different way of looking at a situation. Often in recovery, relapses occur because the core issues are being ignored. Every time those of us who are prone to eating disorders feel overwhelmed, it becomes too tempting to grab the log again. In order to get past the urge to revert, we must discover who we are. In doing so, we begin to recognize our own strength.

Whether I was eating too much, not eating enough or eating and purging through exercise or otherwise, food was a way for me to cope and avoid negative feelings. My disorder was a distraction, something I used to avoid dark feelings and thoughts. Whatever I did with food took my attention away from the situations in my life that were beyond my control and placed it on something more tangible, at least it felt this way initially, but the rules I created for myself were too strict. I was becoming too rigid, and eventually, I got lost in my illness. I became completely numb to the world around me, experiencing only the turmoil and pain of the illness.

Such a magic recovery pill has yet to be invented, literally or metaphorically. Instead, after many years of struggling, I found enough courage to take a first step toward something different, and that was what eventually propelled me onto a path of health. That's all it took, a simple decision to do something different, to try a different path and listen to the small part of myself that had been begging for change. A friend told me to try something, anything different, and at first I thought it would be impossible. I could always go back, she assured me, but I found once I did try something else, something less self-destructive, I didn't want to go back.

Why was it so difficult during those hard years to listen to that voice, the healthy, sensible, rational one that wanted peace? I wish it had been simple, but that's not to say it can't be for some. It took many years of struggling in a whole new way before I could really embrace recovery, however, the decision to try happened in an instant, not unlike my decision to innocently go on a diet in order to gain some control of my life, or so I initially thought.

What I hope to offer here is not so much a step-by-step guide to recovery but more a book of suggestions that anyone can consider at any given time during recovery. We are all unique, so what works for one person might not work for another. There are, however, key issues to address that can potentially help anyone reclaim health. Recovery is not linear or sudden. It doesn't happen overnight. There are ups and downs, but there can be an overall positive trend despite any lows you might face. There's a saying that I and many others have found to be true: *Our worst days in recovery are far better than our best days in the throes of the illness.* Any hardships in recovery are worth it when you get to experience more freedom in recovery.

Eating disorders are not a choice. There are genetic factors, physiological components as well as environmental, emotional and mental aspects to consider. These illnesses are extremely complex, and recovery is not as simple as making *one* decision. Heading into recovery, however, has to begin with intention, a step, no matter how small, in the right direction, a willingness to try something different when you know what you're doing isn't working. A person reaches wellness by making multiple choices on a daily basis, but beginning the journey can be as simple as making a declaration about or a commitment to recovery. Your initial decision must be followed by renewed dedication and actual effort to support the end goal every day. It does get easier, though, and recovery is possible. It just takes patience and a lot of hard work.

* * *

What It's All About

"Count your blessings, not the calories. Weigh your options, not your self-worth. Starve your self-hatred, not your body. Hate the disorder, not yourself." --Anonymous

Understanding some of the contributing factors that led to your illness and getting to know the driving forces behind any unhealthy actions and urges can help you heal. For many individuals, eating disorders are a coping strategy, a logical way to feel safe and in control in a chaotic environment. We are not able to control the world around us, so those of us who are susceptible to eating disorders will often turn to unhealthy and even dangerous behaviors as a way to give ourselves a false sense of control or to distract ourselves from reality.

Throughout your recovery, you must continually ask yourself, *"What is driving these unhealthy thoughts"* or *"What's behind my self-destructive actions?"* Your thoughts and actions are a symptom of something deeper. What is going on in your life now, or what happened in the past, that is pushing you toward engaging in disordered eating? Always ask yourself if you are hungry (physically or emotionally), angry, lonely, or tired (the HALT question common to numerous recovery programs). Ask yourself what additional stresses you are facing, and never be afraid to ask for support.

If you have trouble identifying your emotions, use a chart of emotions or a feelings wheel, such as this one: http://humanemotionschart.com/. Go through a list and ask yourself if the descriptions on any of the emotions on a chart fit with what you are experiencing. Try your best to describe what you are feeling in a journal or diary. Sometimes the mere act of describing what you feel can ease the actual feelings. Try to distinguish between what you are thinking and what you are feeling.

If you have ever lived with dysfunction -- and almost all of us have; whether it's in the family, with friends, a coworker or with a significant other, truly healthy and functional relationships are rare -- chances are that you learned at some point to suppress your feelings. When we shove our feelings down and can't fully express what we feel, we end up behaving differently. Over time, discounting and continually holding in emotions can even lead to feeling physically sick.

Many other conditions, such as anxiety, depression and obsessive-compulsive disorder (OCD), are often comorbid with eating disorders. In fact, quite often, treating an underlying condition such as depression helps with the treatment of an eating disorder. Antidepressants, either synthetic or all-natural (e.g., SAM-e, TravaCor, or St John's wort) can take the edge off the depression and anxiety that often accompany an eating disorder. If possible, work with a therapist, doctor or someone in the medical field who can determine if you are dealing with a mood issue with roots outside your eating disorder. Don't be afraid to try suggested medications if your treatment team feels it's necessary.

Above all, give whatever you try or whatever therapy in which you engage time to have an effect and communicate with your treatment providers how you are feeling along the way. If this is difficult, look into finding a patient's advocate to guide you.

* * *

Nourishment

"There are realities we all share, regardless of our nationality, language, or individual tastes. As we need food, so do we need emotional nourishment: love, kindness, appreciation, and support from others." -- J. Donald Walters

As a note of caution: If you are at a point where *refeeding syndrome* might be a concern, please seek medical attention as soon as possible. Also, eating disorders can affect hormone and electrolyte levels. In general, stress can affect your entire endocrine system, so check in with your general physician or an endocrinologist to make sure you are not experiencing any symptoms related to hormone or endocrine imbalance. Be sure you are following the advice of your recovery team and doctors as you look into these and any other suggestions. Only use what you feel safe using.

Food is fundamental to life, yet many see eating as the most difficult aspect of treatment, however essential it is for recovery. Healing starts with giving your body, including the brain, all it needs to nourish and restore itself, so that it can operate at an optimum level. You have to give yourself permission to eat. Any guilt or shame around eating, no matter what your actual size, must be countered with a reminder that food is a basic right that you deserve and need. Food and nourishment are primarily for the body but also for the mind and the soul, so to speak. And nourishment can take many forms when it comes to how you manage your body.

Moving toward health takes seeing yourself and treating yourself as a whole being. This includes the physical, emotional, mental and even spiritual bodies. We can't expect the cure of a complex illness to be found by focusing on only one aspect of the disorder, however, when it comes to eating disorders, refeeding and getting proper nutrition, no matter what your disorder, is essential. Unfortunately, getting the right nourishment can be one of the scariest steps in the healing process. It's important to keep in mind, though, that the more the body is lacking nutrients, the more distorted thinking generally is.

As an example, a person in the throes of an eating disorder such as anorexia will often feel fat. It seems counterintuitive, but this kind of distortion usually becomes less problematic as weight is restored and the right nutrients are included in the diet. In my own case, I constantly felt fat and uncomfortable in my body during my worst struggles, but when my weight returned to a stable level, I experienced fewer thought distortions and less negative thinking. In fact, the noisy, unhealthy chatter in my head went from being a constant annoyance to eventually slipping into the background to finally giving me peace as I continued to heal.

Whether your pattern includes restricting, binging and purging, or some combination, the ultimate goals in recovery are **restoring health** and **experiencing life again**. These are complementary goals: Progress in one eases the path toward the other. Refeeding can be a difficult step in recovery, and that's why it's safer to have support -- perhaps even in a hospital setting -- when you begin to eat after a long period of restricting or after eating inconsistently. Finding pleasure and enjoyment, even when it comes to eating meals, can happen. For those who believe they are eating too much and feel guilty, look at where these beliefs come from and how realistic they are. As Carmen Cool, MA, LPC says, "Your body, your rules," so aim for both physical and emotional health as much as possible. Sometimes being healthy includes eating a chocolate ice cream cone in the middle of the afternoon with friends or having a second serving of potato chips with your sandwich.

It's not uncommon to have an increased appetite as you begin to nourish your body. In fact, this is normal. Whatever kind of disorder you have, it's so important to make sure you are getting enough protein, healthy fats and carbohydrates during this phase of recovery and that you have the emotional support you need. Cravings can feel scary, but the more you understand them and the more you listen to what the are saying, whether they are emotional or physical needs, the easier it will be to feel at ease when they appear.

I can't stress this enough: *The more support you have from family, friends, therapists, dietitians, nutritionists and/or members of support groups, the better.* You don't have to go through this alone. Knowing we are not alone is a comforting thought, and feeling supported can push us to make the changes we need.

The fear of not being able to stop or control the hunger once you begin eating regularly can be worrisome, but allow yourself time for your body to adjust to the changes and to the different foods you are now consuming. It can take a while for your body to heal and adjust to digesting food regularly again. Your metabolism will probably increase as you eat more and are no longer in a state of starvation. Even if you were not starving before starting your recovery, your body still needs time to get used to consistently receiving and processing the proper nutrients. Please trust me on this -- any uncomfortable feelings will subside. Have faith that the intense hunger will decrease once you get used to eating regular meals.

Honor your hunger, and don't be afraid of it. Acknowledge it and learn that it's OK to eat when you feel hungry. You don't reach a moral high ground or display strength when you restrict and deny yourself what your body needs. On the contrary, it takes courage, conviction and strength to give your body what it desires when you are used to restricting or binging.

Often neglected in discussions about refeeding (or simply changing your diet) is the fact that troubling digestive issues may arise. Digestive enzymes, such as pancreatin and hydrochloric acid, can cause bloating, gas, and that uncomfortable full feeling while they help your body absorb more nutrients. Other symptoms, such as acid reflux, constipation, nausea, excessive hunger, or diarrhea, might require that you seek medical attention. With severe malnourishment, intravenous vitamin drips can be most beneficial. A high-quality multivitamin and mineral tablet – especially one that contains an adequate amount of zinc, a mineral that has been shown to decrease the symptoms of anorexia – is crucial when adequate daily nutrients are missing from the diet. Ultimately, the body is resilient and is able to repair itself when given the chance. Healing is possible. With proper nutrients and an improved mental outlook, complete healing can occur more quickly.

Keep in mind that no single diet will work for everyone. There is no perfect diet, and what is optimal for one person might not be for another. In addition, the diet you settle on now may evolve, and you may find that it changes as your comfort level around eating improves during recovery. Aim for a nutrient-dense diet, but move away from too many rules, especially ones that are too strict. Your diet should be something you create that includes a variety of foods. If you are unsure about what you should be eating, try seeing a nutritionist or dietitian to get you started in the right direction.

Food should nourish both the body and the soul, so to speak. Some people like the idea of intuitive eating, while others like to have a meal plan to use as a guideline. Be sure, though, that meal plans are suggestions only. You should be able to allow any rules around food to be broken when it means you are honoring your physical needs. It's also OK to break rules just because you feel like it, but try to be aware and don't beat yourself up about it afterward. It's your body, and you are allowed to have a say in how and what you eat. This will become more second nature the more you get used to eating a healthy amount.

During meal times, try to make your environment as calm and comfortable as possible with few distractions. Turn off the television, set the table, put your cell phone in the other room, and sit down, so that you can concentrate and be aware of the food you are eating and also be in touch with how you are feeling. Make sure you are addressing any issues that can make meals more stressful and cause an increase in anxiety. Try to make mealtimes stress-free. After meals, use either journaling or distraction to keep from feeling any anxiety related to eating.

Eating out and eating with others can be challenging when you are also dealing with an eating disorder. Not being able to control what you eat and eating in front of others might cause anxiety. Do your best to stay as calm and relaxed as you can. Part of eating with others is the social aspect, so do what you can do focus on enjoying the company you are with. For some, eating with others can actually help them feel more relaxed. Being with others can allow a person to feel safer with trusting that portion sizes are acceptable and with eating in general. Whatever the case, whether you see eating with others as a challenge or an advantage, push yourself to go outside of your comfort zone from time to time.

Fad diets, even those based on scientific findings, do not typically address the emotional aspect of eating. Whether you restricted, binged or purged, make sure you are addressing the underlying emotional issues related to your particular disorder. Always remind yourself that you are deserving and need food to survive. There should be no shame or guilt around eating. Fad diets might give you quick weight-loss results, but they don't teach you how to listen to and trust your body and its needs.

There is nothing wrong with enjoying your food. Many cultures celebrate and use food as a way to socialize. Food can be a way to create warm memories when we learn to get past any disordered thinking around it.

* * *

Body Image

"Beauty is about being comfortable in your own skin. It's about knowing and accepting who you are." -- Ellen DeGeneres

For many, a difficult aspect of recovery is body acceptance. In addition to dealing with any physical changes that might occur during recovery, looking at how you used and perceived your body during your illness can be beneficial. Look at whether you have used your body as protection: to hide or disappear, or as a barrier to others.

Is the dialogue between your mind and your body healthy and positive? How you talk about yourself can shed light on underlying feelings about your overall self-worth. Below is a list of exercises and some ideas designed to help you explore how you feel about your body and help you improve your body image.

I bring up nutrition again here knowing that when people don't give themselves proper nutrition, it affects their thinking. In fact, after World War II, concentration-camp survivors were interviewed and found to have had a warped sense of body image. A body thrown out of balance is unable to perceive reality accurately, and not eating properly can create a vicious cycle of feeling uncomfortable with your body, restricting your intake, and feeling even more discomfort with your body as your perceptions become further skewed. Even though it's easy to understand on an intellectual basis that our size shouldn't determine self worth and value as a human being, accepting this emotionally is harder.

Aim for the center. As you choose life and choose health, a part of you may continue longing to look a certain way. Keep your focus on your recovery as much as possible. Healing doesn't mean going to extremes. The idea that being healthy equals being fat is inaccurate. As you begin to recover, you will find comfort away from the extremes, and instead of seeing every issue only in black and white terms, you might find that there are many potential solutions to any given situation.

Work on your self-esteem. Practice exercises in which you look in mirror and state outright, "I love my body" or "I love myself."

Analyze how this statement makes you feel. Repeat this exercise several times a day for at least 10 days, even if it's difficult, and see if you begin to feel different by the last day. The goal is to eventually accept and appreciate this statement.

Define what beauty means to you. When you look at others, do you see only their outer beauty or is their core more interesting to you? Do you hold yourself to different standards than you do others? How does body size define your self worth, and do you believe it should? What are some ways you can begin to move away from the idea that size is an indicator of value or worth?

Stay away from triggering content. Whether it's an image in a magazine, someone you know who isn't supporting your recovery, or a website that encourages unhealthy behavior, make sure you understand that the beauty industry is trying to sell you products and will encourage you to see yourself as flawed. This is not true. The beauty standard is unrealistic, and often the images used in magazines have been drastically digitally altered. Always remember that you are beautiful the way you are.

Engage in affirmation exercises. Remember that focusing on your body can be another way to distract yourself from feelings or the past. Some good exercises to try around body image include repeating positive affirmations and art therapy. Affirmations include repeating positive statements such as "My body deserves love and respect" or "My body is perfect the way it is, and I honor it in this state."

Create artwork. Art, including drawing, coloring, making collages, sculpting, and painting, engages a different part of your brain than talking or writing does. Sometimes it can be helpful to process what you are feeling through art. It can also help situate you more in the moment, so you are focused on the act of creating rather than getting lost in thoughts around your disorder. Art therapy is designed to reduce stress and can give you a sense of accomplishment. It has actually been shown that creating art changes the brain. It improves brain connectivity and plasticity.

Avoid competition and comparisons. Every single body on this planet is different. Mark Twain once said, "Comparison is the death of joy," and he was right. When we compare, we do so with inaccurate information. We never know the whole story when it comes to someone else. Comparing yourself to others can spiral downward into insecurity. Do your best to keep your focus on yourself and your own goals.

Keep ongoing lists. List the things you appreciate about your body. Write another list of what your body can do and how it serves you. Add to these lists as often as you like.

Forget notions of perfection. As much as possible, move away from the idea that you have to be perfect. The body positive movement has some wonderful ideas around avoiding shaming the body, and this includes your own. As Diane Israel, MA, observes,"Perfection is the core wound of anorexia." She adds, "There is an underlying fear of failure that leads most addicts to seek control through other means."

Don't indulge negativity. Other people's comments can throw you for a loop. If someone makes a negative comment, don't harm yourself because you feel hurt. Never use food or restricting as a punishment. Instead, reach out to friends, write about your feelings or tell the person how his or her comments made you feel. Treat yourself with extra kindness if anything like this occurs and upsets you.

Move away from numbers and the scale. Have a ceremony and toss out your scale or do what members of the Boulder Youth Body Alliance formerly run by Carmen Cool suggest and make a "Yay scale" -- one that's artistically painted or decorated and covers up any numbers with positive affirmations.

* * *

Healing

"At any given moment, you have the power to say, 'This is not how my story is going to end.'" -- Christine Mason Miller

As you begin to heal physically with improved nourishment, you can begin work on overcoming your disorder more fully. Eating disorders are called illnesses for a reason; though classified as mental disorders, they have biological, as well as psychological, features.

Heal the past, and when you are ready, forgive yourself and others. Do this for yourself. Sometimes merely acknowledging what you went through and how difficult it was to endure is enough to begin healing from past traumas. And trauma can be different for everyone. What might seem like no big deal to one person can be incredibly upsetting to another. Processing the situation, healing from the damage and moving forward will make you feel more at ease in general. Express your pain regarding what happened in the past, and let it go. Then, do what you can to focus on the present.

Strategies always available to you include:

Be kind to yourself and to others. As much as possible, observe without judgment. This includes observing the thoughts and feelings you experience, especially those that come up before and after you eat. Ask yourself if the thoughts you have, especially those about yourself, are accurate.

Surround yourself with, and seek out, positive and healthy people. Are there people you admire who lead healthy and well-rounded lives? Who are your role models and who do you look to as an example of a positive role model? Look for role models who are accepting and who embody strength, courage and wisdom.

Notice and care for the child within you. Though you can't go back and change the past, you can provide yourself some comfort and heal from the pain of past events. This includes making sure you are getting the attention, love and care you need now. You can give this to yourself in the form of self-care, or you can ask for help and encouragement from others.

Visualize the future, your future. Imagine yourself healthy and fully able and capable. Jot down a few of your life and long-term goals. Choose these goals over looking a certain way or staying stuck in the disorder. Any time you feel yourself struggling, remind yourself where you want to be. Accept where you are, but keep working on your short- and long-term goals.

Be gentle with yourself. Navigating feelings and learning how to process them can involve bumps in the emotional road. There isn't a specific set of steps to take in order to go through an emotional experience. The main thing is to make sure you are expressing yourself in a healthy way and allowing your feelings to come to the surface. Though it might feel like your sadness or anger will last forever, do as Diane Israel suggests and look at these feelings like you would fluctuations in the weather. A bad storm rolls in, but it eventually passes. It's a temporary situation. You can't control it, but you can control your reactions. You will get through it. Write, scream or cry into a pillow, sing, dance, talk to friends, and do whatever it takes to make sure you are dealing with your emotions safely.

When I read about Jenni Schaefer and her book *Life Without Ed*, I was concerned that she advised people to compartmentalize their thoughts, as if they belonged to a separate entity, in this case "Ed." I strongly believe that our eating disorders are very much a part of ourselves -- something we create and must take ownership of, not something to necessarily fight against; a set of actions and circumstances to understand and from which to learn.

There are times when it feels as if choosing to recover means fighting the urge to harm yourself. This is true, but healing comes from going deeper and addressing the underlying issues, not blaming "Ed" without delving into the whys. The technique of externalization, and using "Ed" (or some other name) to address your disorder, does help to identify the negative thoughts, though, and I fully support that aspect. If it works for you -- whatever works for you, in fact -- then use it.

When you are struggling, it can be difficult to determine whether a given thought is healthy. I don't see anything wrong with labeling a thought "Ed" or any name you like, but, again, I would suggest taking this one step further: Look at why this thought is coming up, and determine how you can address or even counter it in a healthy, positive way. Try writing the thought down first. In a separate column, write out possible reasons why you think this thought arose when it did. Finally, in a third column, see if you can write something positive that opposes or disproves the negative thought.

* * *

<u>Recovery</u>

"I got tired of waiting for the light at the end of the tunnel, so I lit that bitch up myself." -- Anonymous

A lot of information regarding eating disorders exists online and in general, but not all of it is accurate. Be careful to look into research claims and any information that lacks explicit scientific backing. Bloggers might have good intentions, but not all of them are qualified to give advice about eating disorders and especially about recovery. Use your discretion. Mostly, when it comes to advice, use what works for you and discard the rest. When in doubt, check with a professional, your doctor or your therapist, to make sure anything you try is safe.

It can be difficult to say goodbye to an illness or addiction when, as in the case of eating disorders, it serves as a coping strategy. If, however, you are getting the security you need in a healthy way, it becomes easier. The safer you feel, the easier it will be to let go of the disorder.

Some ways to achieve this include:

Write a letter to your illness. Acknowledge how it served you, and then say goodbye to it. Observe how saying goodbye makes you feel.

Be as present and aware as you can in life. There's a strong correlation between your thoughts and your speech and how you feel. The more you can switch your focus away from food, calories and exercise, the more you can allow yourself to be in the moment, and this is a way to temporarily forget your disorder. Aim to avoid triggering statements such as "I feel fat" and instead try to uncover what this symptom means. Often, this translates into feeling uncomfortable. Dig for the cause of the symptom rather than focusing on the symptom itself, and then seek out solutions in healthy ways.

Listen to your body. Do what's sensible, and allow your body its voice. Watch how you talk to yourself and to others. Listen carefully to others who love you and choose your words carefully. When you judge others harshly, also take a look at what is going on for you. Sometimes when we feel uncomfortable with ourselves, we tend to project our own issues onto others.

Be patient with your own mind. Over time, the thoughts that seem so oppressive will start to abate and move to the background. Before long, you will begin to notice that these thoughts will completely disappear for short periods. Soon, the periods of time without the distorted thoughts will stretch into longer and longer segments until you can be more focused on living and less obsessed with what you are eating, how much you are exercising or how your body looks.

Challenge your core beliefs and fears. Keep exploring what rules you create for yourself and why. You set the rules, and you can change them. Some people who have overcome eating disorders explain that they think of their illness like a game in which they create rules by which they force themselves to abide, and, since this is the case for them, they have the power to change or relax the rules. This is your life. You are strong enough to create your own destiny.

I read of one young lady with an eating disorder whose observant mother noted that she slowly began to bend her own rules during her recovery. At first, she wouldn't allow herself to eat outside of her planned meals, but she slowly began to allow herself a little bit extra, a taste of her favorite dish or an extra-thin slice of cake. These "extras" didn't count for her. A few extra bites weren't enough to break her rules, only bend them until she could get to the point where she wasn't unnecessarily constricted by these rules, and could break them, change them or even get rid of them. Start with small steps if a giant leap is too scary at first.

Be grateful of where you are and what you have learned thus far. Keep a gratitude jar and fill it up monthly, weekly or even daily with events or anything for which you are grateful, as little or a big as it may be. Write it on a slip of paper and place it in your gratitude jar.

Whenever you feel you need some encouragement, take out the slips of paper and read them.

* * *

Taking Action

"Vision without action is merely a dream. Action without vision just passes the time. Vision with action can change the world." -- Joel A. Barker

So often when it comes to thinking about recovery and change, it's easy to say or think, "I can't." What would it take to change that to "I can" or "I will"? What is it that holds you back from being where you want to be in your recovery? Is it fear? What is the worst thing that can happen if you choose a different path today? Is it a realistic fear? Keep exploring what it is that holds you back.

There's a saying in AA that goes something like: First it gets easier, then it gets harder. After that it gets really hard. Then it gets easier again, and then you start to live. How can you start living? What kind of activity can you engage in that will help your recovery? What is one thing you can do today to support your recovery?

Some guideposts:

Honesty is crucial when it comes to recovery. You must be honest with yourself and with others. Write out a list of ways in which you hide or don't tell the truth about behaviors or anything related to your eating disorder. In a separate column, write out your truths, things you know are true and would like to share with someone, if not today, one day. Remember, there is no shame in admitting your struggles. Everyone has had them, and it's important to open up about them.

You don't have to be great to be successful. We put so much pressure on people and on ourselves to be the best, to be number one. Instead, be unique. Be you. That's more important. You can do great things when you are healthy, but start by first taking care of yourself and simply being and being OK with that.

Find your identity. You are not your disorder. In my own case, rather than focus on what I was eating or how much I was exercising, I eventually had to turn my attention inward and ask myself what my passions were. I needed to rediscover what I liked and disliked, what my beliefs were and what stirred my emotions. In doing this, I started to better understand how I could move away from the labels that had bound me for so many years. I had to fight the negative thoughts and replace them with positive ones, too. My mantra became, "I am OK and everything will be OK," because I had so many fears and old beliefs running through my mind keeping me from believing that things would ever be even close to OK, let alone good.

Eventually things were good, beautiful at times, but recovery doesn't mean perfection or perpetual happiness. It means you get to participate in the world again and be alive, really living and engaged in life.

Find, and rediscover, your passions. We all have them, and they can become so buried in our sickness that we either forget how important they once were or discount the idea that we can ever reclaim them. Write out and describe your likes and your dislikes that are unrelated to the disorder. Reclaim yourself and your identity apart from the disorder. Think about what movies you like, what books move you and what music resonates with you. Explore what it is about a piece of literature, a movie or a song that makes you like or dislike each. Get to know who you are away from anything related to your eating disorder.

Develop personal mantras. What are your mantras? Find some positive affirmations, however pithy, that encourage and inspire you. Write them out and put them around your home, so that you see them often. Come up with positive mantras to use to counter any negative thoughts that enter your mind, even if it's just thinking, or perhaps saying out loud, "STOP!"

An exercise that can help with reconnecting with who you are and finding your identity is describing yourself in a positive way. What are the characteristics, the features and also the things you do that you are proud of or that you like? Are you kind, compassionate, intense or passionate? What do you like to do for fun? What features do you like on your body? What do you do or what would you like to do for a living? Write all of these out and keep adding to your description.

Explore your own recovery. Create your own path, one that is unique and works for you. Write down your goals. Describe your life in recovery and how you want it to be. When you have a picture in your mind of what you would like your recovery to include, you can begin to take steps to get there.

Join a support group or a recovery forum. Some benefits you get from a group is that you can participate in role playing activities. Sometimes just knowing there are others who have gone through similar situations is helpful. Mostly, though, sharing your thoughts and your struggles can be freeing. It can help you better understand your own illness and how to go about healing from it, and it removes some of the shame we often feel when we think we are alone in our struggles.

Become a mentor or find a recovery buddy. Set an example for others and guide them or give back in some way. You don't have to be 100 percent cured to offer help to someone else in need. You matter. Say to yourself, "I matter." Practice self-love and self-care by acknowledging how strong you are for having come this far. Always give yourself credit for surviving and getting through another day.

A relapse is not failure. This is vital. If you experience a relapse, look at what happened to get you there and look at how you can get back on track as quickly as possible. Ask yourself what was going on before things went awry and if you were under more stress or if you were feeling overwhelmed. Identify what your triggers are and find ways to move forward. Forgive yourself; this is essential. Get the help and support you need, but keep moving forward. Try to see a setback as learning experience, not an excuse to go backward.

It can be reassuring to know that you have the tools you need in order to recover or recover from a relapse. A bad day or a bad week does not mean you are back in the illness completely. You are always one small move away from getting back on track. No matter how hard it seems, you have the strength to do one thing to support your recovery, even if it means calling a friend or a helpline. You are stronger than you may realize.

If I could give only one piece of advice to anyone struggling with an eating disorder, it would be to hold on to the belief that a full recovery is possible. You may not know what that looks like, but the more you can imagine how you want your life to be, the more you can strive to make it happen.

* * *

Family and Friends

"You need a really solid foundation of friends and family to keep you where you need to be." -- Lilly Singh

Addressing family issues can be difficult. If at all possible, look into family-based therapy. Make sure that everyone is getting their needs met. As painful as it can be, sometimes people need to take a break from each other or create strong boundaries in order to maintain their optimal health. Try not to take someone needing space personally. Those who can be there for you will be, and if that's not possible for some, it's OK. Make sure you are getting the support you need from others in that case.

If you are a parent, a friend or a relative of someone who is suffering from an eating disorder, make sure you are also getting the support you need. It can be too easy to focus on the one struggling, but everyone needs support. In addition to the NEDA website, F.E.A.S.T. also has suggestions for those who are supporting others with eating disorders: http://www.feast-ed.org/

* * *

Resources

International suicide helpline:
http://www.suicide.org/international-suicide-hotlines.html

National (U.S.) suicide hotline:

National Suicide Prevention Lifeline 1-800-273-8255

http://www.suicidepreventionlifeline.org/

Organizations:

NEDA National Eating Disorder Association; 1-800-931-2237
https://www.nationaleatingdisorders.org
ANAD national Association of Anorexia Nervosa and Associated
Disorders; (847) 831-3438, http://www.anad.org
NABA National Anorexia & Bulimia Association; (402) 371-0722;
http://www.nabassociation.org
Eating-Disorder.com; (866)-575-8179. Connects people with the
appropriate treatment centers.
F.E.A.S.T. Families Empowered and Supporting Treatment of Eating
Disorders http://www.feast-ed.org/

Books:

Lize Brittin:
Training on Empty

Geneen Roth:
How to Break Free from Compulsive Eating
Feeding the Hungry Heart
When Food is Love

Peggy Claude-Pierre:
The Secret Language of Eating Disorders

Linda Rector Page, N.D., Ph.D.
Healthy Healing

Websites:

https://www.nationaleatingdisorders.org/
http://www.edreferral.com/
http://mentalhelp.net/poc/center_index.php?id=46
www.anred.com

Other types of therapy:

Acceptance and Commitment Therapy (ACT) - A type of psychotherapy that can be used to help people become more aware and accepting of their emotions and life experiences. It is designed to help individuals identify and develop a healthy relationship between their thoughts, emotions and their intellect. This can help reduce anxiety and help treat depression.

Cognitive Behavioral Therapy (CBT) - A form of therapy that teaches individuals to identify and address negative thought patterns and core beliefs that contribute to these negative patterns.   This type of psychotherapy teaches the skills needed to find healthy ways to cope with life situations.

Dialectical Behavioral Therapy (DBT) - This type of therapy combines both cognitive and behavioral methods of treatment as a way to help cope with painful emotions or memories. It relies on mindfulness and emotional regulation and is especially useful in circumstances in which there is conflict. This type of therapy is often beneficial to those who tend to react to stressful situations in extreme ways.

Eye Movement Desensitization and Reprocessing (EMDR) - EMDR is a type of therapy that aids in alleviating the symptoms and emotional distress associated with traumatic life experiences. It is thought to help the brain process past events more effectively and more quickly than talk therapy. During an EMDR session, the therapist will direct an individual to remember emotionally disturbing material in short sequential doses while simultaneously engaging in directed lateral eye movements and sometimes additional external stimuli as well. This is thought to help clients activate their own natural healing process.

Exposure and Response Prevention Therapy (ERP) - This type of psychotherapy is designed to help individuals acknowledge and overcome specific fears and anxiety. A person is gradually exposed to the feared object or situation with the idea that this will eventually have a desensitizing effect. It can also be used to help cope with an eventually overcome both fears and certain urges.

Interpersonal Psychotherapy (IPT) - This type of therapy often helps improve body image and self-esteem. The main focus of IPT is addressing underlying personal problems, such as unresolved grief and role disputes. The therapy is designed to help people learn how to cope with stress and anxiety related to these issues.

#

A special thanks to the following women for their ideas on recovery listed below: Jennifer Crain, Eva Johnson, Lisa Schrump, Erinn Kathleen, Samantha Anne, Caroline Roggenbuck, Diane Israel, Kathleen Ensor and those who chose to remain anonymous.

Suggestion basket:

Whenever possible, have a friend or family member nearby to eat meals with, so that someone can help you be accountable. Have a pre-planned meal plan that includes a lot of variety and options that you can follow each day.

Treat yourself as you would treat others. When facing negative thoughts or anxiety, keep yourself distracted and engaged in things unrelated to food and the eating disorder.

Working the 12 steps helped me take responsibility and stop blaming others. Also, listing three good things every day helps keep my overall outlook positive.

Choose the next best action.

Recovery takes time and hard work. Be patient with yourself.

It takes time for the mind to catch up with the body. Heal your body, and your mind will also heal in time. Also, anticipate some discomfort in recovery.

Think of recovery like climbing a mountain. You will encounter hard, rocky sections that are so difficult, you feel like you want to give up, but if you keep going, you will reach beautiful stretches that are easy to maneuver. There sections are rewarding after struggling to get there. Know that you can keep going in the end.

What was a game changer for me was taking responsibility for changing my choices. It empowered me and gave me the ability to change, even if it sometimes felt uncomfortable. I also received coaching, and that has helped my development and helped me sustain recovery.

Cultivate compassion for yourself and self-love. Work on being aware.

Learn to trust. Know that food is not the enemy. It will allow you to heal. I had to get the right nutrition before I could work on the techniques in therapy that ultimately helped me recover.

Glossary

Acid reflux - Acid reflux is the flow of stomach acid back up into the esophagus, the tube that connects the stomach and the upper throat. Gastroesophageal reflux disease is a more severe form of acid reflux.

Anorexia nervosa - A life-threatening eating disorder characterized by weight loss or abnormally low weight, distorted body image, restricted food intake, fear of gaining weight, and obsessions with weight, food and body.

Art therapy - A model of psychotherapy involving the encouragement of free self-expression through art used in order to encourage self-awareness, reduce stress, manage addictive behaviors and improve self-esteem.

Bloating - An abnormal full feeling and often a distention of the abdominal area usually caused by gas in the intestines, eating too quickly or overeating.

Bulimia - A dangerous eating disorder characterized by eating, usually large quantities of food, and then purging either by vomiting or by other means such as exercise or the use of laxatives.

Digestive enzymes - Proteins that catalyze reactions between other chemicals and ultimately help with the breakdown of food during the digestive process..

Connectivity - (Brain connectivity) A pattern of anatomical links and interactions between distinct units within a nervous system by way of neurons and synaptic connections.

Constipation - Infrequent or difficult to pass bowel movements that may also be hard and dry.

Coping mechanism (or coping strategy) - An action taken or conscious effort applied in order to reduce or better tolerate stress and conflict.

Core beliefs - The main beliefs that generally arise from childhood experiences, personal disposition, cultural or societal influence and are assumed to be true for the person who holds them. They are the essence of how an individual sees himself.

E.D. or ED - Abbreviation for eating disorder.

Feelings chart - A chart, often with images, that helps identify various feelings and helps assist anyone struggling to identify what he is feeling.

Identity - A mental concept of how an individual views herself, including her self-image, individuality, core beliefs and self-esteem. Inner child - The metaphorical child within each human being that represents the neglected, hurt or needy child of the past. In theory, an adult can provide her own inner child the comfort, attention and care she lacked as a child.

Long-term goal - The ambition of a person for a future result, a goal that takes planning and time in order to accomplish.

Mantra - A word, sound or phrase that's repeated frequently in order to aid in focusing attention and concentration in meditation and also one that helps express or change a person's basic beliefs.

Nausea - A sick feeling often accompanied by the urge to vomit.

Plasticity - Neural plasticity refers to the brain's ability to change and form new connections and pathways at any age.

Perfectionism - A disposition that pushes a person to strive, often unrealistically, toward goals without allowing for anything short of the ideal. Failing to reach the often unattainable result often leaves a perfectionist feeling worthless.

Refeeding syndrome - The potentially life-threatening metabolic and clinical changes that occur when a severely undernourished individual is rehabilitated at a rate at which the body can't adapt. Those who are at the greatest risk of developing refeeding syndromes include anorexics, chronic alcoholics, and those with marasmus, chronic malnutrition or kwashiorkor.

Relapse - A decline in an individual's state of health or mental health after a period of improvement.

Self-care - Self-provision and self-maintenance without outside assistance. In recovery, self-care goes one step further in not only making sure basic needs are met but also addressing all needs, emotional and physical.

Short-term goals - The ambition of a person for a desired result in the near future, a goal that takes relatively little planning or time in order to accomplish.

Trigger - A trigger is an event, situation or anything that causes a reaction or response usually related to a memory or past trauma. It can be similar to a flashback that transports a person back to a traumatic past event. Triggers can cause a person to engage in harmful or addictive behaviors in an attempt to reduce the pain and stress around the memories that arise.

Visualization - A cognitive technique used to reduce stress, improve performance and focus attention on specific objects and events. Visualization can include using mental imagery to recreate experience, imagine a specific outcome or direct attention away from specific thoughts or situations.

"Yay scale" - A bathroom scale decorated in such a way as to remove any numbers and to foster positive feelings.

About the Author and Editor

Lize Brittin, a lifelong resident of Boulder, Colorado, has a B.A. in psychology and is the author of the 2012 eBook *Training on Empty,* which chronicles her ferocious struggles with, and recovery from, anorexia nervosa, and co-author of the 2017 book *Young Runners at the Top*. She has been published in LIVESTRONG.com, *Competitor Running*, Thrill Magazine, Fit Cities USA and Boulder County Home and Garden Magazine. Rated one of the top mountain runners in the world in the 1980s, she has worked in careers ranging from teacher to chef to assistant manager of an art gallery, and has also hosted her own radio show and been a guest speaker on KGNU, KRFC, the Women Talk Sports Network and Green Light Radio. She can be found online at http://trainingonempty.blogspot.com, a companion blog to her eponymous memoir.

Kevin Beck, a native of New Hampshire who has extensively traveled the country, has been a professional writer for over 20 years. A former contributing editor and senior writer for *Running Times* magazine, he is the editor of the 2005 training book *Run Strong* and co-author of the recently published book *Young Runners at the Top*. He has also written for *Competitor Running, Men's Fitness, Marathon & Beyond*, the *Concord Monitor*, the *Roanoke Valley Sports Journal*, the New York Road Runners Club, FloridaRunners.com and other online and print health- and fitness-related publications. He has a 1:08 half-marathon and a 2:24 marathon to his credit. Visit him on the Web at www.kemibe.com.

www.ingramcontent.com/pod-product-compliance
Lightning Source LLC
Chambersburg PA
CBHW071144280526
45787CB00003B/1405